THE

MENOPAUSE

WEIGHT LOSS

GUIDE

SARAH JACK

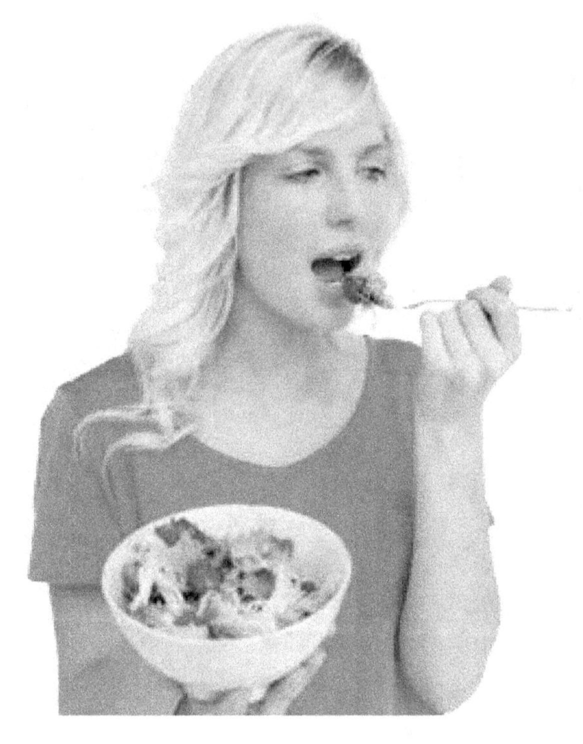

COPYRIGHT

All rights reserved. This book or any portion thereof may not be reproduced or used in any manner whatsoever without the express written permission of the publisher except for the use of brief quotations in a book review.

TABLE OF CONTENTS

Table of Contents

INTRODUCTION

The menopause, a biologically normal process, signals the end of a woman's fertile years. With an average age of 51, it typically affects females between the ages of 45 and 55. A woman's body experiences hormonal changes during menopause that cause her periods to stop and her body to produce less reproductive hormones like estrogen and progesterone.

Menopause symptoms frequently include:

- Hot flashes: Sudden feelings of heat that are frequently accompanied by perspiration and a pounding pulse.

- Hot flashes that happen while you sleep might cause night sweats and disturb your sleep cycle.

- Menstrual cycles start to become erratic before eventually ceasing.

- Reduced estrogen levels might cause vaginal dryness and pain during sexual activity.

- Mood Swings: Hormonal changes might make some women more irritable, depressed, or prone to mood swings.

- Insomnia and other sleep disorders might be prevalent during menopause.

- Libido modifications: Some women report a drop in libido.

- Weight Gain: Hormonal changes, especially in the abdomen, might cause weight gain.

It's significant to remember that each woman has a unique menopause experience. While some women may have severe symptoms that significantly impair their quality of life, others may only experience minor symptoms or none at all.

Causes

Menopause is mostly brought on by aging-related biochemical changes in a woman's body. The following are the main causes of menopause:

- Ovarian Aging: The primary cause of menopause is the ovaries' normal aging. The quantity of eggs in a woman's ovaries is fixed from birth. The quantity of eggs generally decreases as they become older. The synthesis of reproductive hormones like estrogen and progesterone also declines in tandem with this drop in egg production.

- Hormonal Changes: A drop in estrogen and progesterone levels is one of the hormonal effects of ovarian function loss. These hormones are essential for sustaining reproductive health and controlling the menstrual cycle. The typical menopausal symptoms and changes are brought on by the decline in hormone levels.

- Follicle Depletion: The ovaries have organs called follicles that hold developing eggs. Women's follicle counts diminish with age, which affects the body's capacity to release mature eggs for ovulation. The irregular menstrual cycles and eventual cessation of menstruation that take place during menopause are a result of this process.

- Genetic Factors: Genetics can also impact the menopause's date. A woman's chances of going through menopause earlier in life are increased if her mother or older sisters did so. On the other hand, if her family members went through menopause later in life, she might as well.

- Other Factors: The following medical illnesses and procedures can cause menopause to occur earlier than it would naturally:

  ➢ Regardless of a woman's age, oophorectomy surgery results in an abrupt and immediate beginning of menopause.

  ➢ Medical therapies: Chemotherapy and radiation therapy for cancer can harm the ovaries and cause an early menopause.

> Medical Conditions: A number of metabolic illnesses, genetic diseases (such as Turner syndrome), and autoimmune diseases can affect ovarian function and cause early menopause.

- Transition to perimenopause: Hormonal changes and erratic menstrual periods occur during the perimenopausal years, or the years before menopause. This phase is marked by fluctuating estrogen levels, which might cause menopausal symptoms to start to appear. Although the exact time varies, perimenopause commonly begins in a woman's late 30s to early 40s.

It's crucial to remember that every woman will eventually go through menopause as a result of a normal and physiologic process as she ages. Understanding the underlying causes can aid women in navigating this transition more skillfully, despite the fact that the symptoms and experiences can differ greatly.

Consulting a healthcare professional is advised if you have particular menopause-related worries or inquiries.

Complications

Due to the hormonal alterations and physiological changes that take place during this phase, menopause can result in a number of difficulties and health hazards. The following are a few typical issues and health considerations:

- Osteoporosis: As estrogen levels fall after menopause, bone density may also decline, raising the risk of osteoporosis. Bones that are brittle and frail and more prone to fractures are symptoms of osteoporosis. Fractures can seriously affect mobility and general health, which is a serious worry, especially for postmenopausal women.

- Cardiovascular Disease: Estrogen protects against cardiovascular disease by encouraging healthy blood vessel activity and controlling cholesterol levels. The risk of cardiovascular disease, such as heart disease and stroke, rises as estrogen levels fall after menopause. During this stage, maintaining a healthy lifestyle is essential for controlling cardiovascular risk factors.

- Vaginal Atrophy and Pain: Lower estrogen levels can cause vaginal atrophy, which is characterized by the thinning, dryness, and irritation of the vaginal walls. This may result in discomfort, pain during sex, and a higher risk of vaginal infections.

- Urine Incontinence: Modifications to the muscles and tissues of the pelvic floor may cause urine incontinence or an increase in the frequency of urination. This may have an effect on a woman's quality of life and call for management techniques.

- Mood Changes and sadness: Hormonal changes during menopause may cause irritation, mood swings, and a higher risk of sadness or anxiety. Neurotransmitters in the brain that affect mood are regulated by hormones.

- Sexual Health Changes: Due to hormonal changes and the physical discomfort brought on by vaginal dryness, some women experience changes in their sexual desire and satisfaction.

- Weight Gain and Metabolic fluctuations: Hormonal fluctuations can affect body composition and metabolism, which makes managing weight more difficult.

- Cognitive Changes: Some women have "menopausal brain fog," or problems with memory, focus, and cognitive function, during the menopause. Research is still being done to determine the precise connection between menopause and cognitive abnormalities.

- Increased Risk of Specific Cancers: Hormonal changes during menopause may have an impact on the risk of specific cancers, including breast and ovarian cancer. Menopause and cancer, however, have a complicated link that can change depending on things like genetics and lifestyle.

- Sleep Disorders: Hot flashes and night sweats, two frequent menopause symptoms, can interfere with sleep cycles and cause sleep disorders.

It's crucial to remember that not all women will suffer these issues; in fact, some people may experience a relatively easy menopause transition. Maintaining a healthy lifestyle that includes regular exercise, a balanced diet, weight control, and stress reduction is crucial to managing any issues and lowering health risks. Getting medical assistance and direction from healthcare specialists might help you manage menopause-related issues if you're exhibiting major symptoms or worries.

HRT, or hormone replacement therapy, is one method for treating menopausal symptoms. To treat symptoms including hot flashes, vaginal dryness, and mood swings, synthetic hormones are used to replace the diminishing hormones. HRT, however, has advantages and disadvantages, therefore using it should be discussed with a healthcare professional.

Menopausal symptoms can also be controlled by making lifestyle changes such adhering to a nutritious diet, obtaining regular exercise, managing stress, and getting adequate sleep. It is advised to speak with a healthcare professional for advice on the best course of action for your particular circumstance if you're going through menopause and feeling a lot of discomfort.

WEIGHT LOSS

Weight loss is the process of consciously reducing body weight, frequently in order to enhance fitness, appearance, or health. It often entails a mix of dietary adjustments, increased physical activity, and occasionally behavioral changes. When it comes to losing weight, keep in mind the following important factors:

- Diet: Effective and long-lasting weight loss depends on a balanced, nutrient-rich diet. Observe the following guidelines:

  - Caloric Deficit: You must consume less calories each day than you expend in order to lose weight. You can do this by cutting back on your calorie intake or by getting more exercise to burn more calories.

  - Focus on entire, nutrient-dense meals including fruits, vegetables, lean meats, whole grains, and healthy fats when eating healthfully. Reduce your intake of processed foods, sweet drinks, and high-calorie snacks.

> Portion Control: Watch your portions to prevent overeating. Use measuring cups and food scales as tools to help you determine portion sizes precisely.

> Eat mindfully by chewing each bite thoroughly and paying attention to your hunger and fullness indicators. This may aid in reducing calorie intake.

- Physical Activity: By raising your energy expenditure and enhancing your general fitness, regular exercise is essential for weight loss. To help burn calories and build muscle, combine aerobic exercises (such walking, jogging, and swimming) with strength training (with weights or resistance bands).

- Lifestyle Changes: Making long-term lifestyle changes is frequently necessary for successful weight loss.

> Being consistent is essential. Compared to intensive diets or exercise routines, gradual and consistent modifications are more likely to provide long-lasting improvements.

> Behavioral Modifications: Identify emotional or behavioral triggers that may lead to overeating or the development of harmful habits. Create coping mechanisms for stress, boredom, or emotional eating.

> Prioritize obtaining enough good sleep because it helps control hormones that affect metabolism and hunger.

- Hydration: Drinking plenty of water can promote overall health and aid in controlling hunger. Feelings of thirst can occasionally be confused with hunger.

- Accountability and Support: Having a support network, including friends, family, or a weight loss organization, can offer inspiration, encouragement, and accountability.

- Professional Advice: If you have particular health issues, it's a good idea to speak with a doctor or certified dietitian before making major dietary or exercise changes. They can offer you individualized guidance based on your requirements and medical background.

- Set realistic expectations and keep in mind that losing weight is a gradual process. To prevent harming your health or metabolism, aim for a sustainable rate of weight loss (usually 0.5 to 2 pounds per week).

- Long-Term Maintenance: Losing weight is only one stage of the process. Diet, exercise, and lifestyle choices need to be continually monitored in order to maintain a healthy weight.

Keep in mind that each person is unique, so what works for one person might not work for another. Finding a weight loss strategy that is secure, practical, and in line with your unique needs and tastes is crucial. Consider getting advice from a licensed dietician or fitness expert if you're unsure of where to begin.

BENEFITS OF WEIGHT LOSS DURING MENOPAUSE

Losing weight during menopause can have numerous positive effects on one's physical and mental health. Some of the main benefits are as follows:

- Reduced Cardiovascular Risk: Losing weight can assist in reducing the risk of cardiovascular conditions like heart disease and stroke. Due to hormonal changes that put menopausal women at more risk for various ailments, keeping a healthy weight can benefit heart health.

- Better Bone Health: Being overweight increases the risk of osteoporosis and fractures by placing additional stress on the bones. You can lessen this stress and enhance your bone health by decreasing weight, especially in light of the fact that menopause's lowered estrogen levels contribute to the loss of bone density.

- Improved Joint Health: Shedding pounds helps ease strain on joints, especially weight-bearing joints like the knees and hips. Joint pain can be lessened, and mobility can be increased, as a result.

- Better Blood Sugar Control: Weight loss can enhance insulin sensitivity and regulate blood sugar levels, lowering the risk of type 2 diabetes and improving the management of pre-existing diabetes.

- Hormonal Balance: Retaining a healthy weight can help to keep hormone levels more in check. Losing weight may assist with menopausal symptoms including mood swings and hot flashes.

- Better Mood and Self-Esteem: Successful weight loss can elevate self-esteem and body image, resulting in an increase in general mental health and a decreased risk of anxiety or despair.

- Improved Sleep Quality: Being overweight can make sleep disturbances worse, therefore losing weight will improve sleep quality.

- Decreased Risk of Specific malignancies: Weight loss can help reduce the risk of specific malignancies, such as breast and endometrial cancer. Weight gain is linked to greater levels of several hormones that can raise the chance of developing cancer.

- Relief from Joint Pain: Losing weight can ease joint pain and discomfort, which is especially helpful for women who are dealing with joint problems during menopause.

- Overall Physical Fitness: Losing weight can boost functional ability, stamina, and physical fitness, making daily tasks easier to do.

- Better Sexual Health: Losing weight can improve sexual health by increasing self-confidence and easing physical discomfort, such as joint pain or shortness of breath when exercising.

- Long-Term Health Benefits: Preventing the development of chronic illnesses that may be made worse by excess weight by maintaining a healthy weight throughout menopause can benefit your long-term health.

Always keep in mind that losing weight should be done in a sustainable and healthy manner. Extreme workout routines or crash diets can be damaging to your body, particularly during menopause. Before making big adjustments to your diet or exercise regimen, it's crucial to concentrate on slow, steady development and to speak with a healthcare professional or qualified dietitian.

MENOPAUSE WEIGHT LOSS DIET

Essential nutrients should be the main focus of a menopause weight reduction diet while a calorie deficit is created to encourage weight loss. However, it's critical to establish a well-balanced and long-lasting strategy that promotes general health and attends to the specific nutritional requirements that emerge during menopause. An overview of a menopausal diet for weight loss is provided below:

- Select Nutrient-Dense Foods: Make a point of selecting foods that are high in nutrients while being low in empty calories. Point out the following:

    - Include lean meats, chicken, fish, eggs, beans, lentils, tofu, and low-fat dairy products among your sources of protein.

    - Brown rice, quinoa, whole wheat, oats, and whole-grain bread are examples of whole grains to choose from. These deliver both fiber and slowly digesting carbohydrates.

> Include sources of healthy fats such as avocados, nuts, seeds, and olive oil in your diet. These fats aid in satiety and general well-being.

> Fruits and veggies: For a range of vitamins, minerals, and antioxidants, chow down on colorful fruits and vegetables.

- Observe Portion Sizes: To prevent overeating, pay close attention to portion control. To determine the proper serving sizes, use instruments like measuring cups, food scales, and visual references.

- Maintain Hydration: Drink lots of water all day long. Drinking plenty of water can promote general health and aid in appetite control.

- Control your carbohydrate intake by sticking to complex carbs that provide you long-lasting energy and limiting your intake of processed meals and refined sugars.

- Include fiber: Foods high in fiber, such as whole grains, fruits, vegetables, and legumes, can help you feel full and improve digestion.

- Limit your intake of processed meals, sugary drinks, and high-sugar snacks because they can cause weight gain and have a poor effect on your general health. **6.

- Plan balanced meals that combine lean protein, healthy fats, complex carbohydrates, and an abundance of veggies.

- Choose Your Snacks Wisely: If you need a snack, go for Greek yogurt, nuts, seeds, hummus-topped vegetables, or fruit.

- Mindful Eating: Make an effort to savor each bite, consume food slowly, and be aware of hunger and fullness signs.

- Stay Active: Include regular exercise in your daily routine. To support weight loss and general fitness, integrate strength training with cardio exercises.

- Prioritize protein: Eating enough protein will help you maintain lean muscle mass and support your metabolism while you're trying to lose weight.

- Control Stress: Stress has an impact on both weight reduction and general health. Include stress-reduction practices like yoga, deep breathing, meditation, or enjoyable hobbies.

- Consult a professional before making large dietary or exercise changes. A trained dietician or healthcare specialist should be consulted. They can offer you individualized advice depending on your dietary requirements, tastes, and state of health.

- Set Achievable and Realistic Goals: Set attainable and realistic goals for weight loss. For long-lasting benefits, target a steady weight loss of between 0.5 and 2 pounds per week.

Keep in mind that losing weight should be done in a method that promotes your general health and wellbeing. Methods of rapid or excessive weight loss might be harmful, particularly during menopause. Concentrate on developing a long-term, sustainable healthy lifestyle.

EXERCISE AND MENOPAUSE

Menopause is a natural biological process marking the end of a woman's reproductive years. It typically occurs in the late 40s to early 50s, and it brings about hormonal changes, particularly a decline in estrogen levels. These hormonal shifts can lead to various physical and psychological symptoms, including weight gain, bone density loss, mood swings, and decreased muscle mass. Exercise has emerged as a crucial factor in managing and mitigating the effects of menopause. In this comprehensive exploration, we delve into the relationship between exercise and menopause, examining the physiological and psychological benefits, suitable exercise modalities, and considerations for women during this life stage.

- **Physiological Benefits of Exercise During Menopause:**

Weight Management:

Menopause often coincides with weight gain, especially around the abdominal area. Regular exercise helps manage weight by burning calories and improving metabolism. Aerobic exercises, such as brisk walking, jogging, or swimming, are effective for weight control.

Bone Health:

The decline in estrogen during menopause is associated with decreased bone density. Weight-bearing exercises, like walking, running, and resistance training, stimulate bone formation, enhancing bone density and reducing the risk of osteoporosis.

Cardiovascular Health:

Estrogen plays a protective role in cardiovascular health. As its levels decrease during menopause, the risk of heart disease increases. Regular cardiovascular exercise, including aerobic activities, helps maintain heart health, lower blood pressure, and improve circulation.

Muscle Mass and Strength:

Menopausal women often experience a decline in muscle mass and strength. Resistance training, involving weights or resistance bands, can counteract this loss by promoting muscle development, improving metabolism, and enhancing overall strength.

- **Psychological Benefits of Exercise During Menopause:**

Mood Regulation:

Hormonal fluctuations during menopause can contribute to mood swings and increased stress. Exercise triggers the release of endorphins, neurotransmitters that act as natural mood lifters. Engaging in regular physical activity can reduce symptoms of anxiety and depression.

Improved Sleep Quality:

Many menopausal women experience disruptions in sleep patterns. Regular exercise has been linked to improved sleep quality. Activities like yoga or moderate aerobic exercise can promote relaxation and contribute to better sleep.

Cognitive Function:

Hormonal changes during menopause may affect cognitive function. Exercise has been shown to have positive effects on cognitive health, including enhanced memory and cognitive flexibility. Both aerobic exercise and activities that challenge the brain, such as dance or certain sports, contribute to cognitive well-being.

- **Suitable Exercise Modalities for Menopausal Women:**

Aerobic Exercise:

Activities like brisk walking, jogging, cycling, or swimming are excellent choices for improving cardiovascular health, managing weight, and boosting mood. Aim for at least 150 minutes of moderate-intensity aerobic exercise per week.

Resistance Training:

Incorporating resistance training 2-3 times per week can help maintain and build muscle mass. This can include weightlifting, bodyweight exercises, or the use of resistance bands. Focus on major muscle groups, such as legs, arms, and core.

Yoga and Pilates:

These mind-body exercises emphasize flexibility, balance, and strength. They can be particularly beneficial for menopausal women, addressing both physical and mental well-being. Additionally, these exercises often incorporate relaxation techniques, promoting stress reduction.

Balance and Flexibility Exercises:

Menopausal women may experience changes in balance and flexibility. Activities like tai chi or specific balance exercises can help prevent falls and improve overall stability.

Interval Training:

High-intensity interval training (HIIT) can be effective for weight management and cardiovascular health. Short bursts of intense activity followed by periods of rest or lower intensity can boost metabolism and improve fitness.

- **Considerations and Precautions:**

Consultation with Healthcare Professionals:

Before starting a new exercise regimen, especially for women with existing health conditions, it is crucial to consult with healthcare professionals. This ensures that the chosen exercises are safe and appropriate for individual health profiles.

Adaptation to Individual Fitness Levels:

Exercise programs should be tailored to individual fitness levels and preferences. Gradual progression is essential to avoid injury and allow the body to adapt to increased physical activity.

Nutritional Support:

Adequate nutrition is vital during menopause, and exercise can increase nutritional requirements. Menopausal women should ensure they are getting sufficient nutrients, especially calcium and vitamin D for bone health.

Hydration:

Hormonal changes can affect hydration levels. It's important to stay well-hydrated, especially during and after exercise, to support overall health and address potential changes in water balance.

Listen to the Body:

Menopausal women should pay attention to their bodies and make adjustments to their exercise routine as needed. Factors such as fatigue, joint pain, or other discomforts may necessitate modifications to the intensity or type of exercise.

- **Conclusion:**

In conclusion, exercise plays a pivotal role in managing the physiological and psychological aspects of menopause. The numerous benefits, ranging from weight management and bone health to mood regulation and cognitive function, underscore the importance of incorporating regular physical activity into the lives of menopausal women. Tailoring exercise regimens to individual preferences and fitness levels, while considering potential health considerations, ensures a holistic approach to well-being during this transformative life stage. With the right guidance and commitment, exercise can contribute significantly to a positive and healthy menopausal experience.

MENOPAUSE WEIGHT LOSS RECIPES

Turmeric-Spiced Salmon with Quinoa Salad

Ingredients: Salmon fillet, quinoa, cherry tomatoes, cucumber, red onion, turmeric, olive oil, lemon juice, salt, and pepper.

Instructions: Marinate salmon with turmeric, roast, and serve over a bed of quinoa salad tossed with diced vegetables, olive oil, and lemon juice.

Mango Avocado Salsa Chicken

Ingredients: Chicken breast, mango, avocado, red onion, cilantro, lime juice, garlic, salt, and pepper.

Instructions: Grill chicken and top with a refreshing salsa made from diced mango, avocado, red onion, cilantro, lime juice, garlic, salt, and pepper.

Cauliflower and Chickpea Curry

Ingredients: Cauliflower, chickpeas, tomatoes, onion, garlic, ginger, curry powder, coconut milk, cilantro, salt, and pepper.

Instructions: Sauté onion, garlic, and ginger; add cauliflower, chickpeas, tomatoes, curry powder, and coconut milk. Simmer until cauliflower is tender. Garnish with cilantro.

Spinach and Feta Stuffed Turkey Burgers

Ingredients: Ground turkey, spinach, feta cheese, garlic, onion, whole wheat buns, lettuce, tomato.

Instructions: Mix ground turkey with sautéed spinach, feta, garlic, and onion. Form into burgers and grill. Serve in a whole wheat bun with lettuce and tomato.

Lemon Garlic Shrimp with Zoodles

Ingredients: Shrimp, zucchini, garlic, lemon, olive oil, red pepper flakes, salt, and pepper.

Instructions: Sauté shrimp with minced garlic, lemon juice, and red pepper flakes. Serve over spiralized zucchini noodles.

Quinoa and Black Bean Stuffed Peppers

Ingredients: Bell peppers, quinoa, black beans, corn, tomatoes, onion, cumin, chili powder, cheese.

Instructions: Mix cooked quinoa with black beans, corn, diced tomatoes, onion, cumin, and chili powder. Stuff into halved bell peppers, top with cheese, and bake until peppers are tender.

Kale and Berry Salad with Grilled Chicken

Ingredients: Kale, mixed berries, grilled chicken, feta cheese, almonds, balsamic vinaigrette.

Instructions: Toss chopped kale with mixed berries, grilled chicken, crumbled feta, and almonds. Drizzle with balsamic vinaigrette.

Cabbage and Cashew Stir-Fry

Ingredients: Cabbage, cashews, tofu, soy sauce, ginger, garlic, sesame oil.

Instructions: Stir-fry shredded cabbage, cashews, and tofu with soy sauce, ginger, and garlic. Finish with a drizzle of sesame oil.

Salmon and Asparagus Foil Packets

Ingredients: Salmon fillet, asparagus, lemon, dill, garlic, salt, and pepper.

Instructions: Place salmon and asparagus on a foil sheet. Season with lemon, dill, garlic, salt, and pepper. Seal into packets and bake.

Eggplant and Lentil Moussaka

Ingredients: Eggplant, lentils, tomatoes, onion, garlic, cinnamon, nutmeg, olive oil, yogurt.

Instructions: Layer roasted eggplant and cooked lentils with a sauce made from tomatoes, onion, garlic, cinnamon, and nutmeg. Top with a dollop of yogurt.

Tofu and Vegetable Skewers

Ingredients: Tofu, bell peppers, cherry tomatoes, red onion, balsamic glaze.

Instructions: Thread tofu and vegetables onto skewers. Grill until tofu is golden and veggies are tender. Drizzle with balsamic glaze.

Sweet Potato and Black Bean Buddha Bowl

Ingredients: Sweet potato, black beans, quinoa, avocado, lime, cilantro, olive oil.

Instructions: Roast sweet potato, toss with black beans, quinoa, avocado, lime juice, cilantro, and olive oil.

Greek Yogurt and Berry Parfait

Ingredients: Greek yogurt, mixed berries, granola, honey.

Instructions: Layer Greek yogurt with mixed berries and granola. Drizzle with honey.

Mushroom and Spinach Omelette:

Ingredients: Eggs, mushrooms, spinach, feta cheese, olive oil, salt, and pepper.

Instructions: Sauté mushrooms and spinach, pour beaten eggs over, add feta, cook until set, and fold into an omelette.

Pumpkin Seed-Crusted Tilapia

Ingredients: Tilapia fillets, pumpkin seeds, lemon, parsley, garlic, olive oil.

Instructions: Coat tilapia with crushed pumpkin seeds, lemon zest, minced garlic, and parsley. Bake until fish flakes easily.

Quinoa and Vegetable Stuffed Acorn Squash

Ingredients: Acorn squash, quinoa, broccoli, carrots, onion, garlic, thyme, Parmesan cheese.

Instructions: Roast acorn squash halves, fill with a mixture of cooked quinoa, steamed broccoli, carrots, sautéed onion, garlic, thyme, and Parmesan.

Miso-Glazed Eggplant

Ingredients: Japanese eggplant, miso paste, soy sauce, mirin, sesame oil, green onions.

Instructions: Mix miso paste, soy sauce, mirin, and sesame oil. Brush over halved eggplants and broil until caramelized. Garnish with sliced green onions.

Chicken and Vegetable Lettuce Wraps

Ingredients: Ground chicken, lettuce leaves, bell peppers, water chestnuts, soy sauce, ginger, garlic, green onions.

Instructions: Sauté ground chicken with diced bell peppers, water chestnuts, soy sauce, ginger, and garlic. Spoon into lettuce leaves and garnish with sliced green onions.

Cucumber and Avocado Gazpacho

Ingredients: Cucumbers, avocados, tomatoes, red onion, garlic, lime juice, cilantro, vegetable broth.

Instructions: Blend cucumbers, avocados, tomatoes, red onion, garlic, lime juice, cilantro, and vegetable broth. Chill and serve.

Beet and Goat Cheese Salad

Ingredients: Roasted beets, goat cheese, arugula, walnuts, balsamic vinaigrette.

Instructions: Toss roasted beets, crumbled goat cheese, arugula, and walnuts. Drizzle with balsamic vinaigrette.

Lemon Basil Chicken Salad

Ingredients: Grilled chicken, mixed greens, cherry tomatoes, cucumber, red onion, lemon-basil vinaigrette.

Instructions: Arrange grilled chicken over mixed greens, cherry tomatoes, cucumber, and red onion. Drizzle with a lemon-basil vinaigrette.

Spaghetti Squash Primavera

Ingredients: Spaghetti squash, cherry tomatoes, broccoli, bell peppers, garlic, olive oil, Parmesan cheese.

Instructions: Roast spaghetti squash, sauté cherry tomatoes, broccoli, and bell peppers with garlic and olive oil. Toss with cooked squash and top with Parmesan.

Almond-Crusted Cod with Mango Salsa

Ingredients: Cod fillets, almonds, mango, red onion, cilantro, lime juice, olive oil.

Instructions: Coat cod fillets with crushed almonds, bake until golden. Top with a salsa made from diced mango, red onion, cilantro, lime juice, and olive oil.

Brussels Sprouts and Pomegranate Salad

Ingredients: Brussels sprouts, pomegranate seeds, pecans, feta cheese, balsamic vinaigrette.

Instructions: Shred Brussels sprouts, toss with pomegranate seeds, pecans, and crumbled feta. Drizzle with balsamic vinaigrette.

Sesame-Ginger Tofu Stir-Fry

Ingredients: Tofu, broccoli, bell peppers, snap peas, carrots, sesame oil, ginger, soy sauce.

Instructions: Sauté tofu and a mix of colorful vegetables in sesame oil with ginger and soy sauce. Serve over brown rice or cauliflower rice.

Cilantro-Lime Chicken and Quinoa Bowl

Ingredients: Grilled chicken, quinoa, black beans, corn, cilantro, lime juice, cherry tomatoes, avocado.

Instructions: Combine grilled chicken with cooked quinoa, black beans, corn, chopped cilantro, lime juice, cherry tomatoes, and diced avocado.

Spicy Butternut Squash Soup

Ingredients: Butternut squash, vegetable broth, onion, garlic, chili flakes, ginger, coconut milk.

Instructions: Roast butternut squash, sauté onions, garlic, and ginger. Blend with vegetable broth, chili flakes, and coconut milk for a creamy, spicy soup.

Mediterranean Chickpea Salad

Ingredients: Chickpeas, cucumber, cherry tomatoes, red onion, feta cheese, olives, olive oil, lemon juice, oregano.

Instructions: Mix chickpeas with diced cucumber, cherry tomatoes, red onion, feta cheese, and olives. Dress with olive oil, lemon juice, and oregano.

Pistachio-Crusted Cod with Mango Salsa

Ingredients: Cod fillets, pistachios, mango, red pepper, red onion, cilantro, lime juice.

Instructions: Coat cod with crushed pistachios, bake until cooked. Top with a salsa made from diced mango, red pepper, red onion, cilantro, and lime juice.

Stuffed Bell Peppers with Quinoa and Turkey

Ingredients: Bell peppers, ground turkey, quinoa, black beans, corn, salsa, cumin, chili powder, cheese.

Instructions: Cook ground turkey, quinoa, black beans, corn, and salsa. Stuff mixture into halved bell peppers, sprinkle with cumin, chili powder, and cheese. Bake until peppers are tender.

Lemon Garlic Shrimp and Broccoli Stir-Fry

Ingredients: Shrimp, broccoli, garlic, ginger, soy sauce, lemon juice, sesame oil, red pepper flakes.

Instructions: Stir-fry shrimp and broccoli with minced garlic, ginger, soy sauce, lemon juice, sesame oil, and red pepper flakes.

Chia Seed Pudding with Berries

Ingredients: Chia seeds, almond milk, vanilla extract, honey, mixed berries.

Instructions: Mix chia seeds with almond milk, vanilla extract, and honey. Refrigerate overnight and top with mixed berries before serving.

Roasted Brussels Sprouts and Cranberry Quinoa Bowl

Ingredients: Brussels sprouts, quinoa, dried cranberries, pecans, feta cheese, balsamic vinaigrette.

Instructions: Roast Brussels sprouts, toss with cooked quinoa, dried cranberries, chopped pecans, and crumbled feta. Drizzle with balsamic vinaigrette.

Zesty Tofu and Vegetable Skillet:

Ingredients: Extra-firm tofu, bell peppers, zucchini, yellow squash, cherry tomatoes, lime, cilantro, cumin, chili powder.

Instructions: Sauté cubed tofu with sliced bell peppers, zucchini, yellow squash, and cherry tomatoes. Season with lime juice, cilantro, cumin, and chili powder.

Stuffed Acorn Squash with Wild Rice and Pomegranate

Ingredients: Acorn squash, wild rice, pomegranate seeds, pecans, maple syrup, cinnamon.

Instructions: Roast acorn squash halves, fill with cooked wild rice, pomegranate seeds, chopped pecans, a drizzle of maple syrup, and a sprinkle of cinnamon.

Baked Salmon with Dill and Lemon

Ingredients: Salmon fillets, fresh dill, lemon, garlic, olive oil, salt, and pepper.

Instructions: Marinate salmon with chopped dill, minced garlic, lemon juice, olive oil, salt, and pepper. Bake until salmon is cooked through.

Cabbage and Apple Slaw with Grilled Chicken

Ingredients: Shredded cabbage, apples, grilled chicken, Greek yogurt, Dijon mustard, honey, apple cider vinegar.

Instructions: Toss shredded cabbage, diced apples, and grilled chicken. Dress with a mixture of Greek yogurt, Dijon mustard, honey, and apple cider vinegar.

Mango-Avocado Quinoa Salad

Ingredients: Quinoa, mango, avocado, red onion, cilantro, lime juice, olive oil, salt, and pepper.

Instructions: Combine cooked quinoa with diced mango, avocado, red onion, chopped cilantro, lime juice, olive oil, salt, and pepper.

Stir-Fried Tofu with Vegetables

Ingredients: Tofu, broccoli, carrots, bell peppers, snow peas, soy sauce, ginger, garlic, sesame oil.

Instructions: Sauté tofu and a mix of colorful vegetables in sesame oil with soy sauce, ginger, and garlic.

Greek Lentil Soup

Ingredients: Lentils, tomatoes, carrots, celery, onion, garlic, oregano, feta cheese.

Instructions: Simmer lentils with diced tomatoes, carrots, celery, onion, garlic, and oregano. Top with crumbled feta before serving.

Peach and Walnut Spinach Salad

Ingredients: Fresh spinach, peaches, walnuts, feta cheese, balsamic vinaigrette.

Instructions: Toss fresh spinach with sliced peaches, chopped walnuts, crumbled feta, and balsamic vinaigrette.

Cauliflower and Turmeric Soup

Ingredients: Cauliflower, turmeric, coconut milk, vegetable broth, onion, garlic, ginger.

Instructions: Cook cauliflower with turmeric, coconut milk, vegetable broth, sautéed onion, garlic, and ginger. Blend until smooth.

Pesto Zucchini Noodles with Cherry Tomatoes

Ingredients: Zucchini, cherry tomatoes, pesto sauce, pine nuts, Parmesan cheese.

Instructions: Spiralize zucchini into noodles, toss with halved cherry tomatoes, pesto sauce, toasted pine nuts, and grated Parmesan.

Tuna and Avocado Lettuce Wraps

Ingredients: Canned tuna, avocado, cucumber, cherry tomatoes, lettuce leaves, lemon juice, olive oil.

Instructions: Mix canned tuna with diced avocado, cucumber, and cherry tomatoes. Spoon onto lettuce leaves, drizzle with lemon juice and olive oil.

Quinoa and Kale Stuffed Bell Peppers

Ingredients: Bell peppers, quinoa, kale, black beans, corn, salsa, cumin, chili powder, cheese.

Instructions: Cook quinoa, sauté kale, black beans, corn, and salsa. Stuff mixture into halved bell peppers, sprinkle with cumin, chili powder, and cheese. Bake until peppers are tender.

Broiled Grapefruit with Honey and Mint

Ingredients: Grapefruit, honey, fresh mint.

Instructions: Slice grapefruit in half, drizzle with honey, broil until edges caramelize. Garnish with fresh mint.

Cucumber and Radish Salad with Yogurt Dressing

Ingredients: Cucumbers, radishes, Greek yogurt, dill, lemon juice, garlic, salt, and pepper.

Instructions: Slice cucumbers and radishes, toss with a dressing made from Greek yogurt, chopped dill, lemon juice, minced garlic, salt, and pepper.

Asparagus and Mushroom Frittata

Ingredients: Eggs, asparagus, mushrooms, onion, garlic, Parmesan cheese, olive oil.

Instructions: Sauté asparagus, mushrooms, onion, and garlic. Pour beaten eggs over, sprinkle with Parmesan, and bake until set.

Green Tea and Berry Smoothie

Ingredients: Green tea, mixed berries, Greek yogurt, spinach, banana, honey.

Instructions: Blend green tea, mixed berries, Greek yogurt, spinach, banana, and honey until smooth.

Chickpea and Artichoke Mediterranean Bowl

Ingredients: Chickpeas, artichoke hearts, cherry tomatoes, cucumber, olives, feta cheese, lemon vinaigrette.

Instructions: Combine chickpeas, artichoke hearts, halved cherry tomatoes, sliced cucumber, olives, and crumbled feta. Drizzle with lemon vinaigrette.

Cauliflower and Chickpea Tacos

Ingredients: Cauliflower florets, chickpeas, taco seasoning, whole wheat tortillas, lettuce, salsa, Greek yogurt.

Instructions: Roast cauliflower and chickpeas with taco seasoning. Fill whole wheat tortillas with the mixture, and top with lettuce, salsa, and a dollop of Greek yogurt.

Sweet Potato and Black Bean Hash

Ingredients: Sweet potatoes, black beans, bell peppers, red onion, cumin, paprika, eggs.

Instructions: Sauté diced sweet potatoes, black beans, bell peppers, and red onion with cumin and paprika. Serve with a fried egg on top.

Broccoli and Quinoa Casserole

Ingredients: Broccoli, quinoa, chicken or vegetable broth, cheddar cheese, Greek yogurt, garlic, onion.

Instructions: Cook quinoa in broth, mix with steamed broccoli, sautéed garlic and onion, and Greek yogurt. Top with cheddar cheese and bake until golden.

Pear and Walnut Salad with Goat Cheese

Ingredients: Mixed greens, pears, walnuts, goat cheese, balsamic vinaigrette.

Instructions: Toss mixed greens with sliced pears, chopped walnuts, and crumbled goat cheese. Drizzle with balsamic vinaigrette.

Quinoa-Stuffed Bell Peppers with Turkey

Ingredients: Bell peppers, ground turkey, cooked quinoa, tomatoes, black beans, corn, taco seasoning, cheese.

Instructions: Brown ground turkey, mix with cooked quinoa, diced tomatoes, black beans, corn, and taco seasoning. Stuff into halved bell peppers, top with cheese, and bake until peppers are tender.

Sesame-Ginger Broccoli Slaw

Ingredients: Broccoli slaw, edamame, sesame oil, soy sauce, ginger, garlic, sesame seeds.

Instructions: Mix broccoli slaw with steamed edamame, a dressing made from sesame oil, soy sauce, minced ginger, and garlic. Sprinkle with sesame seeds.

Caprese Zucchini Noodles

Ingredients: Zucchini noodles, cherry tomatoes, fresh mozzarella, basil, balsamic glaze.

Instructions: Toss zucchini noodles with halved cherry tomatoes, fresh mozzarella balls, and chopped basil. Drizzle with balsamic glaze.

Lemon-Rosemary Grilled Chicken

Ingredients: Chicken breasts, lemon, rosemary, garlic, olive oil, salt, and pepper.

Instructions: Marinate chicken in a mixture of lemon juice, minced rosemary, garlic, olive oil, salt, and pepper. Grill until cooked through.

Mango and Avocado Quinoa Bowl

Ingredients: Quinoa, mango, avocado, cucumber, red onion, lime juice, cilantro.

Instructions: Combine cooked quinoa with diced mango, avocado, cucumber, red onion, lime juice, and chopped cilantro.

Spaghetti Squash with Tomato-Basil Sauce

Ingredients: Spaghetti squash, tomatoes, garlic, basil, olive oil, Parmesan cheese.

Instructions: Roast spaghetti squash, sauté diced tomatoes, garlic, and basil in olive oil. Serve sauce over spaghetti squash, and sprinkle with Parmesan.

Pistachio-Crusted Chicken Tenders

Ingredients: Chicken tenders, pistachios, whole wheat breadcrumbs, Dijon mustard, honey.

Instructions: Coat chicken tenders in a mixture of crushed pistachios, whole wheat breadcrumbs, Dijon mustard, and honey. Bake until golden.

Cucumber and Mint Detox Water

Ingredients: Cucumber slices, fresh mint leaves, lemon slices, water.

Instructions: Combine cucumber slices, fresh mint leaves, and lemon slices in a pitcher of water. Allow to infuse for a refreshing detox drink.

These recipes offer a mix of flavors and textures while prioritizing nutritional balance for menopausal weight loss. Enjoy experimenting with these dishes to discover new and delicious options that align with your health goals.

THANKS   FOR

READING

THIS BOOK.